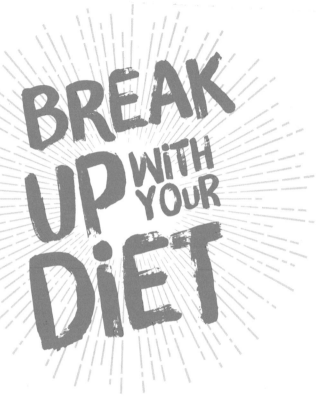

BREAK UP WITH YOUR DIET

A **21-DAY**
Workbook & Journal
for Intuitive Eating

BY GILLIAN ELIZABETH

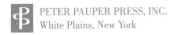

PETER PAUPER PRESS, INC.
White Plains, New York

*To all those looking to feel
free from food:
learn to deeply nourish, accept,
and connect with your body.*

– G E

PETER PAUPER PRESS
Fine Books and Gifts Since 1928

Our Company

In 1928, at the age of twenty-two, Peter Beilenson began printing books on a small press in the basement of his parents' home in Larchmont, New York. Peter—and later, his wife, Edna—sought to create fine books that sold at "prices even a pauper could afford."

Today, still family owned and operated, Peter Pauper Press continues to honor our founders' legacy—and our customers' expectations—of beauty, quality, and value.

TABLE OF CONTENTS

INTRODUCTION

Congratulations! You are now taking the first step toward becoming an intuitive eater. In this workbook and journal you will find motivation, inspiration, and information to help you grow in your personal journey to wellness.

Throughout this journey, you will realize that you can have a healthy relationship with food and a positive body image. Intuitive eating will allow you to be free from restrictions or guilt in regard to eating. This workbook was created to give you the tools to live the best life you can, to free you from your preoccupation with food, and to help you live mindfully.

It takes a minimum of 21 days to form a new habit. After completing this intuitive workbook, mindfulness at the table will be a habit for you. In the beginning, you may be eating one intuitive meal a day, but as time goes on you will find yourself making more intuitive food choices.

Set aside a specific time each day to complete the daily reading and activity in order to finish the workbook in 21 days. Use the prompted daily journal pages to take note of your body's hunger or fullness cues; when + what you eat; and how you feel. Becoming aware through these daily entries will help your eating become more mindful and intuitive. Reading the workbook will provide you with the knowledge and basis of what intuitive eating is but the real understanding comes in when you put the ideas into practice. Not every tip will click right away. Feel free to recommit yourself to 21 days of intuitive eating at a later time or re-read this workbook at your own pace to fully understand the intuitive eating guidelines in this book.

Intuitive eating is a lifestyle—not a diet, although it does require dedication and thoughtfulness. Throughout this program and your life you will be continually rethinking what intuitive eating means to you. You do not need to start with perfection . . . You just have to start.

Break Up with Your Diet is the most powerful tool you can use every day to be healthier, happier, and more in tune with your body, mind, and spirit. I developed this journal after years of trial and error in recovery from an eating disorder. I spent most of my teen years obsessed with the number on the scale and the number of calories I had burned and eaten in a day. I would count my calories, restricting myself, only to "fail" and overeat the next day. The day after that I would over-exercise to burn the extra calories off and devise a new weight goal to start another unrealistic diet—this continued for years. When I discovered intuitive eating I learned to trust my body, stop counting calories, and over-exercising. I started listening to my body instead of my mind, learned what it felt like to be hungry and full (it took me a few months to fully understand my hunger signals), and began to recognize if I wanted to eat due to emotions or true physical hunger.

Do you want to stop . . .
>   . . . obsessing over counting calories?
>   . . . over-exercising?
>   . . . dieting again, and again, and again?
>   . . . worrying that you will never reach your goal weight?

If you said yes to any of the above statements it is a good thing that you picked up this book! Throughout this journal I will teach you the signs of true hunger, how to feel fullness, how to make food choices that truly nourish your body and soul, and how to achieve your ideal weight for life. This journal will set you free in more ways than you think; you will finally be truly living your life! Through my journey I have realized that there are many forms of perfection; you have to allow your body to find the natural weight you are meant to be at and embrace the healthy and powerful being you are. You can tell you have reached your ideal body when you no longer focus your day around when the next meal time is, you totally trust yourself, and you honor your body's cravings—knowing that what it is telling you is what will nourish you the most. Let go of any expectations or ideas about what your intuitive eating journey will look like and begin today!

~Gillian

BREAK UP WITH YOUR DIET

Diets do not work.

It is as simple as that. Yes, some people lose weight, but they also often gain it back. Diets do not work because people are usually losing weight with a target date and weight in mind. Once people have reached their goal weight they do not know what to do. Some people continue on crash course diets and dangerously undereat, while others may slide back into the eating habits they had before.

Eventually, all of these dieters will come to a breaking point—it may take days, weeks, or years. Most diets eliminate whole food groups, revolve around eating every set amount of hours, or require serious tracking of every calorie that you consume. These rules are not sustainable after a long day at work, if you're on vacation, or if you're out with your friends at a dinner party.

Do not buy into lose-weight-fast gimmicks! Diets are temporary. Intuitive eating is a permanent lifestyle.

Results of dieting:
- Irritability
- Inability to psychologically feel full
- Preoccupation with food
- Weight loss followed by weight gain
- Slower metabolism

Results of intuitive eating:
- Sustained weight control
- Avoidance of eating disorders
- Health and happiness!

ACTIVITY OF THE DAY

Throw out or remove any items that may make you tempted to try the next fad diet. This can include magazines, scales (yes, this means you will commit to stop weighing yourself, at least for the next 21 days), tape measures, or clothes you bought for when you reach a certain size. You may want to avoid behaviors that will make you tempted to try dieting again, such as going shopping, reading too many women's magazines, or discussing diet and eating habits.

List the items that you discarded:

....

....

....

....

....

How did that make you feel?

....

....

....

....

....

*I've been on a diet for two weeks and
all I've lost is fourteen days.*
TOTIE FIELDS

BRINGING MiNDFuLNESS TO THE TABLE

*Mindful eating is very pleasant.
We sit beautifully. We are aware of
the people surrounding us. We are
aware of the food on our plates.
This is a deep practice.*

THICH NHAT HANH

Intuitive eating is a skill like any other that requires practice to make perfect. Practicing mindfulness and noticing how the taste of food changes as you become fuller are the goals for today.

ACTIVITY OF THE DAY

Pick one meal to be mindful of during today. Sit at the table with no distractions. That means no cell phone, TV, computer, or book. Before you take a bite of your food, notice the colors and smells. After you take your first bite, notice the texture, flavor, and the thoughts that arise in your head. Chew slowly and notice how the food changes in texture and flavor. Notice when the food does not taste as good anymore—this may be an indicator that your body is satisfied.

How did the exercise go? When, where, and what did you eat? Did you notice anything different about this meal compared to previous meals?

TRUST YOUR GUT—PART 1

Understanding Hunger Levels

How can you tell if you're actually hungry, or if you just want food? There IS a difference. Learning how to tune in to your body and trust your gut takes practice and mindfulness. Your body will give you clues to let you know when you're hungry (versus when you just want food—which might be for a multitude of other emotional or psychological reasons).

Hunger Cues
- A gentle hollow area about the size of your fist
- Stomach growling above your belly button—not below
- Gradual increase in hunger
- Openness to suggestions about food
- Feeling light
- Headache

After you become familiar with these indications of hunger, you'll start to realize and recognize that if you're feeling things quite different from the cues above (such as instant hunger, second-guessing if you are hungry or not, needing one specific food, or being persuaded by commercials or the proximity of tempting restaurants), then that most likely means you are not actually hungry.

Think of your hunger on a scale from 1 to 5. Staying between levels 2 and 4 is optimal for honoring your hunger and satiety cues.

Hunger Levels
1. Do not want to think about food
2. Pleasantly satisfied
3. Neutral
4. Interested in food, hollow area growling
5. All you can think about is food!

When you feel hungry depends on the amount of food last eaten, type of food eaten, and how much activity you have done since eating. The average amount of time it takes for a person to be truly hungry again after a meal is four hours, though it can range between two and six hours depending on your metabolism. A slow metabolism does not mean you will gain weight, it means that you may find yourself intuitively eating fewer times during the day because it takes you longer than average to get hungry.

Understanding Fullness Levels

How can you tell when you're beginning to feel full, satisfied, or if you've gone past fullness and feel stuffed? People feel fullness as a physical sensation. An important part of learning when to stop eating, is tuning in to when you feel satisfied. Satisfaction hovers around level 4 on the fullness scale. Here are some clues to help you become aware of when you are feeling satisfied:

Satisfaction Cues
- Food begins to lose its flavor
- Realization that you could eat more, but it seems unnecessary to do so
- Reflex of leaning back in your chair and taking a breath

Similarly to how you rate your hunger, you can rate your levels of fullness on a scale from 1 to 5.

Fullness Levels
1. Food is bursting with flavor
2. Food tastes good
3. Neutral
4. Completely satisfied, food is losing its flavor
5. Too full, uncomfortable

ACTIVITY OF THE DAY

Start your first day of keeping an intuitive eating journal. Intuitive eating is more about how, why, and what effect food has on your well-being as a whole, as opposed to what food you are consuming and how many calories it has.

Using the journal pages in this book after each daily entry, you will record your body's hunger cues expressed throughout the day. This could include many things such as a growling stomach, headache, tiredness, or feeling light. Write down the times you eat, what you eat, and where your hunger and fullness levels are before and after your meals. You will notice you will be asked to record what you *wanted* to eat versus what you *ended up* eating. This is because many people eat what they feel they should eat rather than what they truly want. Many times when you do this your focus for the rest of the day remains on food and you begin to have cravings because you weren't satisfied at your last meal. In addition, write down *where* you ate. You may find that certain environments promote a more mindful dining experience than others. And of course, don't forget to write how you feel after each meal.

It's also not a bad idea to keep track of any exercise you performed, and how it made you feel, in addition to how many glasses of water you have and how many servings of fruits and veggies. The number of icons that are included on the journal pages aren't meant as recommended quantities, but rather as an easy, visual way for you to keep track and be mindful of these vital nutrients.

As you continue through this workbook, you'll learn more tips about eating intuitively, but for now, today's goal is to just get started! After you've completed your first day of intuitive eating journaling *(see pages 14–15)*, be sure to write about how it went on the opposite page.

How did the first day go?

DATE: M T W Th F S Su

BREAKFAST

Time _____ am/pm _____ Hunger level: **1 2 3 4 5**

Hunger cue: _____

What do I want? _____

What and where did I eat? _____

_____

How do I feel? _____ Fullness level: **1 2 3 4 5**

LUNCH

Time _____ am/pm _____ Hunger level: **1 2 3 4 5**

Hunger cue: _____

What do I want? _____

What and where did I eat? _____

_____

How do I feel? _____ Fullness level: **1 2 3 4 5**

SNACK

Time _____ am/pm _____ Hunger level: **1 2 3 4 5**

Hunger cue: _____

What do I want? _____

What and where did I eat? _____

_____

How do I feel? _____ Fullness level: **1 2 3 4 5**

FRUITS AND VEGGIES:

14

DINNER

Time _____ am/pm   Hunger level: **1 2 3 4 5**

Hunger cue: _____

What do I want? _____

What and where did I eat? _____

_____

_____

How do I feel? _____   Fullness level: **1 2 3 4 5**

_____

SNACK

Time _____ am/pm   Hunger level: **1 2 3 4 5**

Hunger cue: _____

What do I want? _____

What and where did I eat? _____

_____

_____

How do I feel? _____   Fullness level: **1 2 3 4 5**

_____

EXERCISE

Time _____ am/pm

How did I feel before? _____

_____

Activity performed: _____

_____

_____

How do I feel after? _____

_____

WATER: 🥤 🥤 🥤 🥤 🥤 🥤 🥤 🥤

15

TRUST YOUR GUT – PART 2

Part of learning to trust your gut is eating what you really want to eat. If you're standing in the cafeteria line looking at the chicken teriyaki and your mouth begins to water, but instead you choose a salad, you will not feel satisfied. You will end up overeating because you will continue to eat until you eat what you really want.

To get insight into what type of food you are craving, ask yourself "What do I want to eat?" before choosing each meal. You may not have a specific food come to mind, but rather a type of food. Reference these categories to help you clarify what you feel like eating.

- Hearty / Light
- Hot / Cold
- Creamy / Crunchy
- Sweet / Salty
- Flavorful / Mild

There are no "good" or "bad" foods—rather, there are foods that make you *feel good* and foods that make you *feel bad*. When you know that no foods are off limits it's easy to stop eating when you're full because you know you can eat it later when you're hungry.

Food rules of intuitive eating:
NO restricted food
NO guilt
NO foods are labeled as "good" or "bad"

Remember to trust your gut! In the beginning of this journey you will want the foods you've been restricting and that is OKAY. You must allow yourself to eat anything to have a normal relationship with food. You may find yourself eating cookies, cake, and ice cream for almost every single meal. This is part of the process. Many people fear that if they allow themselves to eat any food they desire, they will be out of control and binge on everything.

Typically, this is not the case. The simple act of removing the restriction will take the power away from the food and place it back in your hands, lowering the desire to binge. Think about it this way: If you tell yourself "I can't eat that piece of cake," you will only think MORE about eating the cake! If you tell yourself "I *can* eat that piece of cake," then the less likely it will be that you'll think about eating it.

If you do end up bingeing, cultivate compassion for yourself! Typically you will only binge if your body is extremely malnourished and it needs energy. If you do end up bingeing—see it as a gift. It is an opportunity for you to recognize that something is very out of balance in your body and this journey is your opportunity to restore balance into your life. If you want to have a lifelong healthy relationship with food the hardest part may be trusting your body to tell you what it wants and needs. Over time, your body will develop the ability to guide you when making decisions about timing, content, and size of meals.

ACTIVITY OF THE DAY

Go to the grocery store and buy a variety of foods that you know you enjoy eating. Let yourself eat what you want for an entire day. However, remember to eat when you are hungry and stop when you are satisfied.

Take the first step in faith.
You don't have to see the whole
staircase, just take the first step.
MARTIN LUTHER KING, JR.

BREAKFAST

Time _____ am/pm _____   Hunger level: 1 2 3 4 5

Hunger cue: ....

What do I want? ....

What and where did I eat? ....

....

....

How do I feel? ....   Fullness level: 1 2 3 4 5

....

LUNCH

Time _____ am/pm _____   Hunger level: 1 2 3 4 5

Hunger cue: ....

What do I want? ....

What and where did I eat? ....

....

....

How do I feel? ....   Fullness level: 1 2 3 4 5

....

SNACK

Time _____ am/pm _____   Hunger level: 1 2 3 4 5

Hunger cue: ....

What do I want? ....

What and where did I eat? ....

....

....

How do I feel? ....   Fullness level: 1 2 3 4 5

....

FRUITS AND VEGGIES:

DINNER

Time .... am/pm   Hunger level: **1 2 3 4 5**

Hunger cue: ....

What do I want? ....

What and where did I eat? ....

....

....

How do I feel? ....   Fullness level: **1 2 3 4 5**

....

SNACK

Time .... am/pm   Hunger level: **1 2 3 4 5**

Hunger cue: ....

What do I want? ....

What and where did I eat? ....

....

....

How do I feel? ....   Fullness level: **1 2 3 4 5**

....

EXERCISE

Time .... am/pm

How did I feel before? ....

....

Activity performed: ....

....

....

How do I feel after? ....

....

WATER: 🥛 🥛 🥛 🥛 🥛 🥛 🥛 🥛

HOW TO BOUNCE BACK AFTER A FOOD BINGE

Try to remember a time when you ate past your fullness cues and experienced a food binge. In addition to the obvious long-term effects of overeating such as weight gain, you may have also experienced other side effects such as low self-esteem, stomach pain, guilt, restlessness, boredom, headaches, and even feeling lonely. Did you adopt a destructive "all or nothing" attitude and continue to eat food even though you were no longer hungry? Did you think "Well, I've already messed up, so I might as well mess up some more"? Let me put this attitude into perspective for you. For example, if you accidentally got a small hole in your shirt, would you get out the scissors and make it even bigger just because it already had a small hole in it anyway? I didn't think so.

If you find yourself in a situation where you are overeating or have overeaten, recognize and challenge your thoughts about food. Try to stop thinking in extreme "black and white" or "all or nothing" terms. If you notice you are thinking this way, try to change your thought pattern. Instead of thinking in these "black and white" terms (such as seeing food as good or bad), think about seeing things more in the gray zone. Food is not good or bad—food is energy. Sometimes, you may take in more than you need but it's not as if the food itself is the culprit. The culprit is not tuning in to what your body is really telling you it needs.

Accept that you may have overeaten. The key is to move on! If you fall into feeling guilty for overeating, you will get sucked back into the cycle of undereating, overeating, guilt, repeat. Do not dwell on the fact that you should not have eaten that much. Take note about how your body is feeling. Do you feel sick? Are your pants a little too tight now? The only way to feel better is to let your body digest what you ate and try to be mindful of your fullness level at your next meal. It may be hard to detect when to eat again because your digestion will feel off kilter. In this circumstance ONLY, it may be beneficial to eat exactly four hours after your binge even if you may not feel hungry, instead of skipping any meals.

Use Flow to Combat a Binge

Flow is achieved when you are completely engaged in an activity and lose track of time. These types of activities will be beneficial as exit strategies during or after a binge. There is a multitude of ways to find flow within your day and they will be different for everyone.

Here are a few examples of how to move on after a binge by engaging your mind:

- Watch a movie
- Read a book
- Go for a walk
- Meditate
- Exercise
- Learn something new

ACTIVITY OF THE DAY

Think about activities that fully engage your mind and allow you to nurture yourself without using food as a comfort. Whether it's reading, listening to music, or talking with friends and family, write down a list of these activities that you enjoy. You'll be able to use this as your go-to list if you feel a binge-eating episode coming on.

The true measure of success is how many times you can bounce back from failure.

STEPHEN RICHARDS

DATE:		M	T	W	Th	F	S	Su

BREAKFAST

Time _____ am/pm   Hunger level: 1 2 3 4 5

Hunger cue: ....

What do I want? ....

What and where did I eat? ....

....

How do I feel? ....   Fullness level: 1 2 3 4 5

....

LUNCH

Time _____ am/pm   Hunger level: 1 2 3 4 5

Hunger cue: ....

What do I want? ....

What and where did I eat? ....

....

How do I feel? ....   Fullness level: 1 2 3 4 5

....

SNACK

Time _____ am/pm   Hunger level: 1 2 3 4 5

Hunger cue: ....

What do I want? ....

What and where did I eat? ....

....

How do I feel? ....   Fullness level: 1 2 3 4 5

....

FRUITS AND VEGGIES:

DINNER

Time _____ am/pm   Hunger level: **1 2 3 4 5**

Hunger cue: _____

What do I want? _____

What and where did I eat? _____

_____

_____

How do I feel? _____   Fullness level: **1 2 3 4 5**

_____

SNACK

Time _____ am/pm   Hunger level: **1 2 3 4 5**

Hunger cue: _____

What do I want? _____

What and where did I eat? _____

_____

_____

How do I feel? _____   Fullness level: **1 2 3 4 5**

_____

EXERCISE

Time _____ am/pm

How did I feel before? _____

_____

Activity performed: _____

_____

_____

How do I feel after? _____

_____

WATER: 🥤 🥤 🥤 🥤 🥤 🥤 🥤 🥤

EMOTION-, DEPRIVATION-, AND HUNGER-DRIVEN EATING

People turn to food for many reasons. Once you learn the difference between emotion-, deprivation-, and hunger-driven eating you can assess your own motivations for eating and try to align yourself with an intuitive hunger-driven eating lifestyle.

Emotion-Driven Eating

This type of eating is driven by thoughts and feelings that are unresolved. Food acts as a distraction to push down these thoughts. Ultimately, by avoiding these emotional issues by distracting yourself with food, the cycle of emotion-driven eating will only continue.

Characteristics of emotion-driven eating:
- Internal cues do not drive eating
- Continuing to eat past fullness
- Feeling soothed by eating
- Triggered by your thoughts (not your stomach)
- Eating is a distraction
- Feelings of guilt after eating

Tips to avoid emotion-driven eating:
- Work toward increasing intuition to honor your hunger cues
- Psychotherapy
- Learn to name and feel your feelings
- Meditation (to increase self-awareness)
- Keep a record of satiety and meal times
- Develop healthy personal boundaries

Deprivation-Driven Eating

Deprivation-driven eating is caused by restricting certain foods or food groups. This can be caused by dieting, psychological disorders, or economic or medical reasons. By continuing to deprive yourself of one thing or another, you will not feel satisfied and will constantly feel undernourished—both physically and often mentally.

Characteristics of deprivation-driven eating:
- History of dieting and weight cycling
- History of limited access to food
- Food categorized as good or bad

Tips to avoid deprivation-driven eating:
- Work toward eating in response to internal hunger cues
- Do not restrict any food
- Stop labeling food as good or bad
- Make food available at all times
- Psychotherapy

Hunger-Driven Eating

This type of intuitive eating is a response to internal hunger and it is stopped in response to satiety and fullness cues. Nutritional information is utilized as a way to support your lifestyle—not as a way to form dietary restrictions and rules.

Characteristics of hunger-driven eating:
- Free from worry or preoccupation with food and body
- Eating for enjoyment and health to support lifestyle
- Eating in response to internal cues most of the time

ACTIVITY OF THE DAY

Take time during the day to assess why you are eating. Write down the reasons you ate without judgment toward yourself. Eat without guilt and move on.

DATE: M T W Th F S Su

BREAKFAST

Time .... am/pm .... Hunger level: **1 2 3 4 5**

Hunger cue: ....

What do I want? ....

What and where did I eat? ....

....

....

How do I feel? .... Fullness level: **1 2 3 4 5**

....

LUNCH

Time .... am/pm .... Hunger level: **1 2 3 4 5**

Hunger cue: ....

What do I want? ....

What and where did I eat? ....

....

....

How do I feel? .... Fullness level: **1 2 3 4 5**

....

SNACK

Time .... am/pm .... Hunger level: **1 2 3 4 5**

Hunger cue: ....

What do I want? ....

What and where did I eat? ....

....

....

How do I feel? .... Fullness level: **1 2 3 4 5**

....

FRUITS AND VEGGIES:

DINNER

Time .... am/pm   Hunger level: **1 2 3 4 5**

Hunger cue: ....

What do I want? ....

What and where did I eat? ....

....

....

How do I feel? ....   Fullness level: **1 2 3 4 5**

....

SNACK

Time .... am/pm   Hunger level: **1 2 3 4 5**

Hunger cue: ....

What do I want? ....

What and where did I eat? ....

....

....

How do I feel? ....   Fullness level: **1 2 3 4 5**

....

EXERCISE

Time .... am/pm

How did I feel before? ....

....

Activity performed: ....

....

....

How do I feel after? ....

....

WATER: 🥤 🥤 🥤 🥤 🥤 🥤 🥤 🥤

EATING INTUITIVELY "CHECK-IN"

So it's Day 7 of learning how to become an intuitive eater. Let's check in to see how you're doing!

In the past 6 days you've begun to:

- Practice mindfulness when you eat.
- Trust your gut by tuning in to your hunger and fullness levels.
- Pay attention to satisfaction cues.
- Learn what you really want to eat.
- Think about food as energy—not as good or bad.
- Align yourself with hunger-driven eating.

What's important to remember is that learning how to eat intuitively takes practice and patience. When you begin eating intuitively you may find yourself eating all of the foods you restricted yourself from or shamed yourself for eating. This is a healthy part of the process. During this journey, you may notice some foods do not provide you with lasting energy, and over time you will be less likely to eat those foods and opt for more satisfying foods.

Continue to remind yourself of the basics:

- Before you eat, continue to assess your body's cues.
- Eat when you are hungry.
- If you are hungry, try to figure out what you want to eat. Do you want to taste sweet, bitter, sour, savory, or salty?
- When you have picked out a meal or snack, sit down, be mindful, and enjoy what you are eating. Be fully present for your meal.
- Stop eating when you are satisfied.

ACTIVITY OF THE DAY

An important part of intuitive eating is getting in touch with your body. Yoga is a wonderful tool to help you achieve body and mental awareness because it utilizes both physical movement and meditation. It helps bring you into the present moment—allowing you to be more mindful of your hunger and satisfaction cues.

Take a yoga class today! If you're new to yoga, find a beginner class, or look online for a beginner tutorial video—there are lots of great resources out there. Enjoy this gift to yourself!

I never had a policy; I have just tried to do my very best each and every day.

ABRAHAM LINCOLN

DATE:	M	T	W	Th	F	S	Su

BREAKFAST

Time _____ am/pm .... Hunger level: 1 2 3 4 5

Hunger cue: ....

What do I want? ....

What and where did I eat? ....

....

....

How do I feel? .... Fullness level: 1 2 3 4 5

....

LUNCH

Time _____ am/pm .... Hunger level: 1 2 3 4 5

Hunger cue: ....

What do I want? ....

What and where did I eat? ....

....

....

How do I feel? .... Fullness level: 1 2 3 4 5

....

SNACK

Time _____ am/pm .... Hunger level: 1 2 3 4 5

Hunger cue: ....

What do I want? ....

What and where did I eat? ....

....

....

How do I feel? .... Fullness level: 1 2 3 4 5

....

FRUITS AND VEGGIES:

DINNER

Time _____ am/pm   Hunger level: 1 2 3 4 5

Hunger cue: _____

What do I want? _____

What and where did I eat? _____

_____

_____

How do I feel? _____   Fullness level: 1 2 3 4 5

_____

SNACK

Time _____ am/pm   Hunger level: 1 2 3 4 5

Hunger cue: _____

What do I want? _____

What and where did I eat? _____

_____

_____

How do I feel? _____   Fullness level: 1 2 3 4 5

_____

EXERCISE

Time _____ am/pm

How did I feel before? _____

_____

Activity performed: _____

_____

_____

How do I feel after? _____

_____

WATER: 🥛 🥛 🥛 🥛 🥛 🥛 🥛 🥛

QUENCH YOUR THIRST THE INTUITIVE WAY

As with foods, drinks are not considered good or bad within this lifestyle. Similarly to food choices, you can tune in to what will make you feel refreshed and choose that beverage.

By the time people feel thirsty, they may already be slightly dehydrated. Dehydration may present with symptoms of dry eyes, headache, sluggishness, dry skin, nausea, or constipation. Drinking water at regular intervals can help you to avoid dehydration while still giving you the freedom to choose other beverage options throughout the day.

Beyond the basic H_2O, you can always opt for infusing your water with a variety of flavors. Try out this recipe or any of the pairings on the opposite page.

Infused Water Recipe

Ingredients:

 2 limes
 1 lemon
 1 small cucumber
 10 mint leaves
 4 cups cold water
 Ice cubes (optional)
 1 liter pitcher

Directions:

Rinse limes, lemon, cucumber, and mint leaves. Thinly slice the limes, lemon, and cucumber. Place the slices in the pitcher. Tear mint leaves off of the stem and place in the pitcher. Add the water and ice cubes to fill the pitcher. Refrigerating the water for two to six hours will infuse the flavors together. Enjoy!

Infusion Pairings

blueberry + pomegranate

orange + lemon + lime

pineapple + mint

mint + cucumber + lemon

mint + lavender + lime

blackberry + lime

strawberry + kiwi + cucumber

ginger + lemon

ACTIVITY OF THE DAY

Try creating your own infused water recipe. You could add berries, cucumbers, lemons, or your favorite fruits and herbs to your water to satisfy your creativity and thirst. Share your recipe with other intuitive eaters by using #breakupwithyourdiet.

Your body holds deep wisdom.
Trust in it. Learn from it. Nourish it.
Watch your life transform and be healthy.
BELLA BLEUE

DATE: M T W Th F S Su

BREAKFAST

Time _____ am/pm   Hunger level: 1 2 3 4 5

Hunger cue: ....

What do I want? ....

What and where did I eat? ....

....

....

How do I feel? ....   Fullness level: 1 2 3 4 5

....

LUNCH

Time _____ am/pm   Hunger level: 1 2 3 4 5

Hunger cue: ....

What do I want? ....

What and where did I eat? ....

....

....

How do I feel? ....   Fullness level: 1 2 3 4 5

....

SNACK

Time _____ am/pm   Hunger level: 1 2 3 4 5

Hunger cue: ....

What do I want? ....

What and where did I eat? ....

....

....

How do I feel? ....   Fullness level: 1 2 3 4 5

....

FRUITS AND VEGGIES:

DINNER

Time _____ am/pm _____ Hunger level: **1 2 3 4 5**

Hunger cue: ....

What do I want? ....

What and where did I eat? ....

....

....

How do I feel? .... Fullness level: **1 2 3 4 5**

....

SNACK

Time _____ am/pm _____ Hunger level: **1 2 3 4 5**

Hunger cue: ....

What do I want? ....

What and where did I eat? ....

....

....

How do I feel? .... Fullness level: **1 2 3 4 5**

....

EXERCISE

Time _____ am/pm

How did I feel before? ....

....

Activity performed: ....

....

....

How do I feel after? ....

....

WATER: 🥤 🥤 🥤 🥤 🥤 🥤 🥤 🥤

H. A. L. T. BEFORE YOU EAT

The H.A.L.T. method is a basic tool used by many within the psychology field. It has many applications and can be used by everyday people in their everyday lives. It is a way to check in with yourself before you make any potentially harmful, self-destructive decisions. Basically, if you feel a self-destructive behavior coming on, this technique encourages you to halt, take a moment, and ask yourself "Am I Hungry, Angry, Lonely, or Tired?" before acting. The theory is that if one of these physical or emotional conditions is not being met, you can isolate which one it is and address it directly. When it's framed in the context of overeating, or simply eating when you're not really hungry, it helps you to zone in on why you're motivated to eat.

Throughout this journey, you're developing the skills to listen to your intuition. Pay attention to the hunger cues that are outlined in Day 3. If your body is truly seeking food nourishment because you are hungry, follow those intuitions. But make sure that you're not eating as a result of being angry, lonely, or tired. Try to think of alternatives to eating that can address these conditions instead.

Mindfulness can be summed
up in two words: pay attention.
Once you notice what you're doing,
you have the power to change it.

MICHELLE BURFORD

H

Am I hungry? To become in tune with the feeling of hunger, try to eat meals more slowly. If you are still hungry after you eat, wait 20 minutes and reassess your hunger level.

A

Am I angry? When people are angry, they tend to crave a release. Instead of turning to food, try exercising, taking a shower, cleaning, or singing loudly to music.

L

Am I lonely? Food can seem comforting in the face of loneliness. Instead of eating, try calling a friend, watching a movie, or spending time with your pet.

T

Am I tired? Hunger signals can be hard to interpret when you are tired, which makes it hard to know when to eat. Instead of eating, take a nap, meditate, or treat yourself to a relaxing bath.

ACTIVITY OF THE DAY

Before every bite of food today stop and ask yourself "Am I hungry, angry, lonely, or tired?" Do not judge yourself for eating when you are not hungry. At this stage you want to be able to identify your reason for eating.

DATE: M   T   W   Th   F   S   Su

BREAKFAST

Time _____ am/pm   Hunger level: **1 2 3 4 5**

Hunger cue: ....

What do I want? ....

What and where did I eat? ....

....

....

How do I feel? ....   Fullness level: **1 2 3 4 5**

LUNCH

Time _____ am/pm   Hunger level: **1 2 3 4 5**

Hunger cue: ....

What do I want? ....

What and where did I eat? ....

....

....

How do I feel? ....   Fullness level: **1 2 3 4 5**

SNACK

Time _____ am/pm   Hunger level: **1 2 3 4 5**

Hunger cue: ....

What do I want? ....

What and where did I eat? ....

....

....

How do I feel? ....   Fullness level: **1 2 3 4 5**

FRUITS AND VEGGIES:

DINNER

Time _____ am/pm   Hunger level: 1 2 3 4 5

Hunger cue: _____

What do I want? _____

What and where did I eat? _____

_____

How do I feel? _____ Fullness level: 1 2 3 4 5

_____

SNACK

Time _____ am/pm   Hunger level: 1 2 3 4 5

Hunger cue: _____

What do I want? _____

What and where did I eat? _____

_____

How do I feel? _____ Fullness level: 1 2 3 4 5

_____

EXERCISE

Time _____ am/pm

How did I feel before? _____

_____

Activity performed: _____

_____

_____

How do I feel after? _____

_____

WATER: 🥛 🥛 🥛 🥛 🥛 🥛 🥛 🥛

41

SATISFACTION AND EXIT STRATEGIES

Earlier in the workbook (on Day 3), you learned about paying attention to various satisfaction cues—one of which was noticing when food begins to lose its flavor. This is an extremely helpful tool for realizing and assessing your overall fullness levels. But what if you're having trouble figuring out when exactly this occurs during your meal?

Try this:

Each time you sit down to eat something, rate the first bite of your food on a scale from 1 (being bland) to 10 (being mouth-watering). This will make it easier to identify when your food loses its flavor—at this point you are likely satisfied enough to stop eating.

Additional tips to help you feel more satisfied:

- Give yourself unconditional permission to eat.
- Sit down and eat in a designated area.
- Do not eat when distracted.
- Use a medium-sized plate. Psychological studies support the fact that when you eat off of a smaller plate than usual, you can feel more satisfied with the same amount of food. (This is not to suggest eating portions that are too small however.)
- Make your meal visually appealing.
- Eat the best part first as opposed to saving the best part for last. You will find satisfaction sooner.
- Do not be afraid to leave food on your plate.
- Savor your food.

Another helpful tool when it comes to honoring your satisfaction cues and fullness levels is implementing exit strategies.

Exit strategies can be used to stop eating when you are satisfied but everyone around you is still eating, or if you tend to mindlessly continue to eat if food is left on your plate. In these ways we send a signal to ourselves that our meal is finished.

Some exit strategies include:
- Putting your napkin over your food
- Brushing your teeth
- Having plans to do something right after your meal
- Starting to do the dishes

ACTIVITY OF THE DAY

Figure out which exit strategy will be best for you to utilize when you are at work, home, a restaurant, or a dinner party. Brushing your teeth at a restaurant is not very realistic so you may want to plan a different strategy, or come up with your own personal exit strategies. Write them below:

DATE: M   T   W   Th   F   S   Su

BREAKFAST

Time _____ am/pm _____ Hunger level: **1 2 3 4 5**

Hunger cue: _____

What do I want? _____

What and where did I eat? _____

_____

How do I feel? _____ Fullness level: **1 2 3 4 5**

LUNCH

Time _____ am/pm _____ Hunger level: **1 2 3 4 5**

Hunger cue: _____

What do I want? _____

What and where did I eat? _____

_____

How do I feel? _____ Fullness level: **1 2 3 4 5**

SNACK

Time _____ am/pm _____ Hunger level: **1 2 3 4 5**

Hunger cue: _____

What do I want? _____

What and where did I eat? _____

_____

How do I feel? _____ Fullness level: **1 2 3 4 5**

FRUITS AND VEGGIES:

44

DINNER

Time .... am/pm   Hunger level: 1 2 3 4 5

Hunger cue: ....

What do I want? ....

What and where did I eat? ....

....

....

How do I feel? ....   Fullness level: 1 2 3 4 5

....

SNACK

Time .... am/pm   Hunger level: 1 2 3 4 5

Hunger cue: ....

What do I want? ....

What and where did I eat? ....

....

....

How do I feel? ....   Fullness level: 1 2 3 4 5

....

EXERCISE

Time .... am/pm

How did I feel before? ....

....

Activity performed: ....

....

....

How do I feel after? ....

....

WATER: 🥛 🥛 🥛 🥛 🥛 🥛 🥛 🥛

INTUITIVE EATING AT WORK OR SCHOOL

Congratulations! You have made it halfway through this workbook! Remember to release your expectations about what you or your journey should look like at this point. Today's theme is intuitive eating at work or school. I understand that it can be difficult to eat intuitively when you have set lunch breaks. People typically fall into one of two categories when they are faced with regimented hours. The first category is those who eat out of habit. You are used to eating breakfast, lunch, snack, and dinner at the same time every single day so that is what you do whether you are hungry or not. On the other side of the spectrum, there are those who well up with anxiety trying to pencil into their agenda exactly when and what they will eat. I hate to break it to you, but neither of these approaches will allow you to honor your body. Begin to treat each break as an opportunity to honor yourself by checking in with your body. You may find that the lunch you packed is not satisfying enough, or you may find you would feel more nourished by moving your body with a yoga class or a walk around the block in the fresh air. Here are some tips that can promote intuitive eating at work or school:

- Pack your lunch in the morning instead of the night before because you will have a better idea of what you may feel like eating that day. If circumstances allow, the ideal solution would be to come home for lunch.

- Keep snacks like nuts or protein bars handy in your locker, backpack, or drawer.

- Buy your lunch.

- Drink water throughout the day. People can misinterpret thirst for hunger.

- Consider changing your breakfast time if you find you are not hungry or ravenous when lunchtime rolls around.

ACTIVITY OF THE DAY

Treat yourself and go out for lunch today. Make sure you think about what you want to eat before wandering around a food court. What colors, flavors, textures, or temperature are you drawn to? Let that guide you to a food that your body really, truly wants.

Nourishing yourself in a way that helps you blossom in the direction you want to go is attainable, and you are worth the effort.

DEBORAH DAY

DATE: M T W Th F S Su

BREAKFAST

Time .... am/pm .... Hunger level: **1 2 3 4 5**

Hunger cue: ....

What do I want? ....

What and where did I eat? ....

....

....

How do I feel? .... Fullness level: **1 2 3 4 5**

....

LUNCH

Time .... am/pm .... Hunger level: **1 2 3 4 5**

Hunger cue: ....

What do I want? ....

What and where did I eat? ....

....

....

How do I feel? .... Fullness level: **1 2 3 4 5**

....

SNACK

Time .... am/pm .... Hunger level: **1 2 3 4 5**

Hunger cue: ....

What do I want? ....

What and where did I eat? ....

....

....

How do I feel? .... Fullness level: **1 2 3 4 5**

....

FRUITS AND VEGGIES:

DINNER

Time _____ am/pm _____   Hunger level: 1 2 3 4 5

Hunger cue: ....

What do I want? ....

What and where did I eat? ....

....

....

How do I feel? ....   Fullness level: 1 2 3 4 5

SNACK

Time _____ am/pm _____   Hunger level: 1 2 3 4 5

Hunger cue: ....

What do I want? ....

What and where did I eat? ....

....

....

How do I feel? ....   Fullness level: 1 2 3 4 5

EXERCISE

Time _____ am/pm ....

How did I feel before? ....

....

Activity performed: ....

....

....

How do I feel after? ....

....

WATER: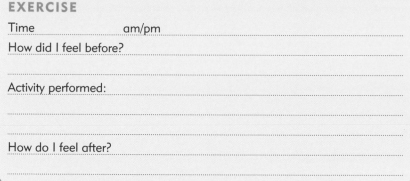

ACCEPT AND RESPECT YOUR BODY

As you continue to eat intuitively you will become more in tune with your body. Happiness is not a size, but a feeling of appreciation for yourself. This happiness will come in steps when you allow yourself to celebrate small gains in your intuitive eating and in your life. Savor the personal victories before celebrating with others—you do not need anyone else's approval.

Acceptance is heavily tied to honesty—one of the most difficult aspects of this lifestyle. Be honest with yourself about how you feel and the reason you are eating. If you are not in a positive state of mind, ask yourself what you can do to shift your mind-set. It does not serve you to eat for emotional reasons.

Being mindful of your emotions, stressors, sleep, and wellness all tie into this lifestyle. Understanding your mental and physical state will help you listen to your intuition. Being mindful is a skill that should be practiced daily, and you can hone this skill by utilizing other resources such as yoga and guided meditation.

More often than not, we get caught in a trap of comparing ourselves and our bodies to others, which inevitably leads us further away from self-acceptance and self-respect. Comparisons are a negative thought pattern. Instead, you can use affirmations to realize your beauty and uniqueness. They can be practiced in front of a mirror, in your head, or spoken out loud, but the most important thing is to practice them often and with intention. Lead yourself on a journey to accept and respect your body using the affirmations on the following page.

Affirmations:

I am enough.

The food I eat energizes and nourishes my body.

I feel happy, healthy, and strong in my body.

I am in tune with my body's nutritional signals.

I am confident knowing that I respect and accept my body.

I love myself.

I am the creator of my own well-being.

I trust myself to listen to my body.

Tip:

You can create your own affirmations by identifying your negative self-talk and transforming it into positive affirmations. Write down all of the reasons you love yourself. Read often.

ACTIVITY OF THE DAY

Develop a daily self-care practice for increasing self-love. This can include: scheduling quiet time for yourself in the morning or after work, going for a massage, taking a bubble bath, meditating, getting rid of social media accounts or magazine subscriptions that foster negative comparisons, using affirmations, or joining an exercise class.

Love yourself first, and
everything else falls in line.
LUCILLE BALL

DATE: M T W Th F S Su

BREAKFAST

Time _____ am/pm _____ Hunger level: **1 2 3 4 5**

Hunger cue: _____

What do I want? _____

What and where did I eat? _____

_____

_____

How do I feel? _____ Fullness level: **1 2 3 4 5**

_____

LUNCH

Time _____ am/pm _____ Hunger level: **1 2 3 4 5**

Hunger cue: _____

What do I want? _____

What and where did I eat? _____

_____

_____

How do I feel? _____ Fullness level: **1 2 3 4 5**

_____

SNACK

Time _____ am/pm _____ Hunger level: **1 2 3 4 5**

Hunger cue: _____

What do I want? _____

What and where did I eat? _____

_____

_____

How do I feel? _____ Fullness level: **1 2 3 4 5**

_____

FRUITS AND VEGGIES:

DINNER

Time _____ am/pm _____ Hunger level: **1 2 3 4 5**

Hunger cue: ....

What do I want? ....

What and where did I eat? ....

....

....

How do I feel? .... Fullness level: **1 2 3 4 5**

....

SNACK

Time _____ am/pm _____ Hunger level: **1 2 3 4 5**

Hunger cue: ....

What do I want? ....

What and where did I eat? ....

....

....

How do I feel? .... Fullness level: **1 2 3 4 5**

....

EXERCISE

Time _____ am/pm _____

How did I feel before? ....

....

Activity performed: ....

....

....

How do I feel after? ....

....

WATER: 🥤 🥤 🥤 🥤 🥤 🥤 🥤 🥤

GENTLE NUTRITION

Gentle nutrition means eating to honor your body by feeding it the nutrients it needs to thrive without forcing yourself to make choices based solely on nutritional information. This being said, not all food is created equal. Each type of food serves a different purpose in your body and you will notice the effects based on what you are consistently eating.

There are six essential nutrients that everyone needs to have in order to achieve and maintain a healthy lifestyle—proteins, carbohydrates, fats, vitamins, minerals, and water. Remember, it's not necessarily about counting grams to meet specific nutritional daily guidelines, but rather it's about paying attention to how you feel when you consume these various essential nutrients. Your body will tell you what it needs—you just have to learn how to listen to it. Let's take a closer look at the three types of nutrients that provide you with energy: proteins, carbohydrates, and fats.

Proteins

Protein plays an important role in the body to build, repair, and maintain healthy cells. Protein is made up of amino acids. There are about 20 amino acids, nine of which are referred to as essential amino acids because the body cannot make them itself—they must be consumed through diet. There are two types of proteins: complete and incomplete. Complete proteins contain all of the essential amino acids. Incomplete proteins do not have all of the essential amino acids, but you can pair incomplete proteins together to make up a complete protein.

On the opposite page are some examples of complete and incomplete proteins and complementary pairings of incomplete proteins that make up complete proteins when combined.

Complete Proteins	Incomplete Proteins

Complete Proteins
- Fish
- Hemp seeds
- Chia seeds
- Chicken
- Eggs
- Quinoa
- Milk
- Yogurt
- Beef

Incomplete Proteins
- Nuts
- Most seeds
- Most grains
- Legumes
- Vegetables

Incomplete Protein Pairings That Make Up Complete Proteins
- Rice and beans
- Hummus and whole-grain pitas
- Whole-wheat bread and peanut butter

Our body is precious. It is our vehicle for awakening. Treat it with care.

BUDDHA

Carbohydrates

Carbohydrates provide your body with energy and are broken into two different groups: simple carbohydrates and complex carbohydrates. Simple carbs provide your body with quick energy—and as you may have guessed, include various kinds of simple sugars (i.e. sucrose, fructose, glucose, etc.). You may find that eating sugary refined foods gives you a small burst of energy, but will not provide you with long-lasting fullness. You may feel that you need to eat again soon after your meal, or you may feel very lethargic. Complex carbohydrates include starches and fiber—both will provide you with longer-lasting energy than a simple carb. There is A LOT of information out there about the do's and don'ts of consuming various carbs, but one thing to keep in mind is that it's always good to strive to eat carbs that are in their most natural forms, rather than those that have been refined over and over again (like the refined starches found in white food products such as bread, bagels, and pasta). Fruits and vegetables are great sources of carbohydrates because they also contain other nutrients and fiber that are beneficial to your body's well-being. Below are just some examples of different food sources of carbohydrates.

Simple Carbohydrates
- Fruit juice
- Honey
- Maple syrup
- Molasses
- Table sugar

Complex Carbohydrates
- Chick peas
- Broccoli
- Wheat
- Peas
- Barley
- Corn
- Lentils
- Leafy greens
- Oats
- Carrots
- Potatoes

Fats
Fat has gotten a bad rap over the years, but some fats are essential nutrients. The essential fats include monounsaturated fats, polyunsaturated fats, and omega-3 fatty acids (which are technically polyunsaturated fats but are often distinguished because of their additional health benefits). All of these fats are known to boost brainpower, curb hunger, and contribute positively to your heart health.

Saturated and trans fats are not considered essential to function. Saturated fats are mainly found in animal products. Some foods that contain saturated fat include red meat, egg yolks, and whole milk dairy products. Trans fats are typically found in foods which contain preservatives such as fast foods, doughnuts, fried foods, cookies, and some margarines. On the opposite page are some examples of essential sources of fats.

Monounsaturated and Polyunsaturated Fats, and Omega-3 Fatty Acids

- Avocados
- Almonds
- Sunflower seeds
- Olive oil
- Tuna
- Mackerel
- Walnuts

- Peanut butter
- Olives
- Sesame seeds
- Flaxseed
- Salmon
- Seaweed
- Hemp seeds

ACTIVITY OF THE DAY

Make a list of what foods make you feel satisfied for a long time after consumption. Some days you may find a certain food more satisfying than another. Also record foods that make you feel good after you eat them, not basing this on taste, but on the absence of heartburn or other unpleasant body sensations. Remember this is not a restriction, it is an observation.

DATE: M T W Th F S Su

BREAKFAST

Time _____ am/pm   Hunger level: **1 2 3 4 5**

Hunger cue:

What do I want?

What and where did I eat?

How do I feel?   Fullness level: **1 2 3 4 5**

LUNCH

Time _____ am/pm   Hunger level: **1 2 3 4 5**

Hunger cue:

What do I want?

What and where did I eat?

How do I feel?   Fullness level: **1 2 3 4 5**

SNACK

Time _____ am/pm   Hunger level: **1 2 3 4 5**

Hunger cue:

What do I want?

What and where did I eat?

How do I feel?   Fullness level: **1 2 3 4 5**

FRUITS AND VEGGIES:

DINNER

Time .... am/pm   Hunger level: **1 2 3 4 5**

Hunger cue: ....

What do I want? ....

What and where did I eat? ....

....

....

How do I feel? ....   Fullness level: **1 2 3 4 5**

....

SNACK

Time .... am/pm   Hunger level: **1 2 3 4 5**

Hunger cue: ....

What do I want? ....

What and where did I eat? ....

....

....

How do I feel? ....   Fullness level: **1 2 3 4 5**

....

EXERCISE

Time .... am/pm

How did I feel before? ....

....

Activity performed: ....

....

....

How do I feel after? ....

....

WATER:

THE INS AND OUTS OF DIGESTION

Becoming attuned to recognize what foods your body craves, digests well, and reacts to can be a challenge. An important tool in figuring this out is focusing not on what goes *in*, but what comes *out*. Noticing your bowel movements can help you understand what foods your body requires for optimal digestion.

By noticing your stool, you may realize that you do not fully absorb the nutrients of certain foods. The amount of time it takes for food to pass through your body can vary greatly for each individual and can depend on what you ate and even how well you chewed your food (smaller pieces of food will generally be digested more quickly). Roughly, it can take an average of anywhere between 24 to 48 hours for food to fully pass through your body. You can refer back to your intuitive eating journal to get a sense of how long some of your foods have taken to digest. Recognizing which foods you consistently do not digest properly can help you adjust your food choices in the future.

Bowel movements can indicate a deficiency or excess of elements within your diet, acting as a monitor for your health. For example, if your bowel movement floats, it may be an indicator of too much fat in the diet or that you're not properly absorbing fats. Knowing your "normal" frequency and color of bowel movements can help you keep your health in check.

In Day 13 you learned about carbohydrates—one of which is fiber. In addition to providing our bodies with energy, fiber also greatly helps to regulate our bowels. Because it is usually tough and rough (think dark leafy greens, bran, seeds, etc.), the body does not completely break it down like it does other food sources. Simply put, big, bulky fiber is going to bulk up your stool, making it easier to pass through—avoiding constipation.

Not only does fiber help keep you regular, but it can also lower your cholesterol, regulate blood sugar levels, help you maintain your weight, and even lower your risk of heart disease.

Here are some sources of foods high in fiber:

- Barley
- Beans
- Seaweeds
- Seeds
- Whole grains
- Vegetables
- Oats
- Lentils
- Brown rice
- Nuts
- Fruits

ACTIVITY OF THE DAY

Ponder Your Poop!

Keep track of your bowel movement(s) and write down the times of day you went, and the characteristics of your movements. Pay attention to the texture, color, size and make note of it here. Has the food you consumed 48 hours ago passed through your body? (You may want to consider continuing to track your bowel movements as it can provide much insight into what types of food you digest well or not.)

DATE: M T W Th F S Su

BREAKFAST

Time .... am/pm .... Hunger level: **1 2 3 4 5**

Hunger cue: ....

What do I want? ....

What and where did I eat? ....

....

How do I feel? .... Fullness level: **1 2 3 4 5**

....

LUNCH

Time .... am/pm .... Hunger level: **1 2 3 4 5**

Hunger cue: ....

What do I want? ....

What and where did I eat? ....

....

How do I feel? .... Fullness level: **1 2 3 4 5**

....

SNACK

Time .... am/pm .... Hunger level: **1 2 3 4 5**

Hunger cue: ....

What do I want? ....

What and where did I eat? ....

....

How do I feel? .... Fullness level: **1 2 3 4 5**

....

FRUITS AND VEGGIES:

DINNER

Time .... am/pm .... Hunger level: **1 2 3 4 5**

Hunger cue: ....

What do I want? ....

What and where did I eat? ....

....

....

How do I feel? .... Fullness level: **1 2 3 4 5**

....

SNACK

Time .... am/pm .... Hunger level: **1 2 3 4 5**

Hunger cue: ....

What do I want? ....

What and where did I eat? ....

....

....

How do I feel? .... Fullness level: **1 2 3 4 5**

....

EXERCISE

Time .... am/pm

How did I feel before? ....

....

Activity performed: ....

....

....

How do I feel after? ....

WATER: 🥛 🥛 🥛 🥛 🥛 🥛 🥛 🥛

63

Rx: SLEEP

Even just one single sleepless night can lead you to choose high-calorie and high-fat foods. Lack of sleep can disturb the hormones that regulate appetite, and this disruption can lead to weight gain. To improve your sleep, try to go to bed when you are feeling tired and wake up when you are fully rested. Of course, this can be a challenge if you're working full-time, but try to get a consistent amount of sleep each night. Over time, your body may become in tune with natural light so that when it becomes dark you will rest, and when the sun is shining again you will awaken peacefully.

Recommendations for a good night's sleep:
- Set a time to go to bed and wake up every day.
- Do not view screens within an hour of going to bed.
- Rub sesame, vetiver, cedarwood, or lavender oil onto your feet before bedtime.
- Use a diffuser to infuse your room with calming essential oils such as chamomile or lavender.
- Drink chamomile tea or warm milk with a pinch of nutmeg.
- Avoid taking naps as this can disrupt the equilibrium of the body and mind.
- Take a bubble bath.
- Practice yoga, yoga nidra, or meditation before bed to help reduce anxiety and tension.
- Make a bedtime ritual which you follow daily to prepare your body for sleep.

ACTIVITY OF THE DAY

Think about how many hours of sleep are necessary for you to function optimally and write it below. Based on this observation, try to create and write down a routine that will allow you to get this many hours of sleep each night. Start tonight!

*Sleep is that golden chain that ties
health and our bodies together.*

THOMAS DEKKER

DATE: M T W Th F S Su

BREAKFAST

Time .... am/pm .... Hunger level: **1 2 3 4 5**

Hunger cue: ....

What do I want? ....

What and where did I eat? ....

....

....

How do I feel? .... Fullness level: **1 2 3 4 5**

....

LUNCH

Time .... am/pm .... Hunger level: **1 2 3 4 5**

Hunger cue: ....

What do I want? ....

What and where did I eat? ....

....

....

How do I feel? .... Fullness level: **1 2 3 4 5**

....

SNACK

Time .... am/pm .... Hunger level: **1 2 3 4 5**

Hunger cue: ....

What do I want? ....

What and where did I eat? ....

....

....

How do I feel? .... Fullness level: **1 2 3 4 5**

....

FRUITS AND VEGGIES:

DINNER

Time _____ am/pm   Hunger level: **1 2 3 4 5**

Hunger cue:

What do I want?

What and where did I eat?

How do I feel?   Fullness level: **1 2 3 4 5**

SNACK

Time _____ am/pm   Hunger level: **1 2 3 4 5**

Hunger cue:

What do I want?

What and where did I eat?

How do I feel?   Fullness level: **1 2 3 4 5**

EXERCISE

Time _____ am/pm

How did I feel before?

Activity performed:

How do I feel after?

WATER: 🥤 🥤 🥤 🥤 🥤 🥤 🥤 🥤

STOP PREVENTATIVE EATING

When you know you have a jam-packed day ahead with very little opportunity to sit down and eat, you may slip from intuitive eating practices. Try not to eat a "preventative" meal to stop yourself from getting hungry during the day, but instead continue to listen to the satiety signals your body sends you. If you are not hungry and eat preventatively your body will not utilize this energy and it will be stored in the body as fat. This is because your body is still breaking down and utilizing the energy from the last meal you ate. Your mind may try to convince you otherwise and you may begin to fear that you will not have enough. Remember what F.E.A.R. stands for: False Evidence Appearing Real. Your body knows how to function in circumstances when you may not have access to food for an extended period of time. When you do get a chance to eat, your body may send signals that it is ravenous and needs a large meal. Try eating half and waiting a few minutes to see if you are still hungry.

Tip:
Pack almonds, a protein bar, or any other protein-rich, non-perishable food item you like to eat into your briefcase, purse, car, desk drawer, or backpack. These convenient snacks can help stave off the lethargic feelings you may experience when your body begins to use its energy reserves to fuel your day.

No matter how much it gets abused,
the body can restore balance. The first
rule is to stop interfering with nature.

DEEPAK CHOPRA

ACTIVITY OF THE DAY

Create your go-to list of protein-rich, satisfying snack foods that you can use as a resource when you know you have a busy day coming up and you'll need to avoid preventative eating.

DATE: M   T   W   Th   F   S   Su

BREAKFAST
Time .... am/pm ....   Hunger level: 1 2 3 4 5
Hunger cue: ....
What do I want? ....
What and where did I eat? ....
....
....
How do I feel? ....   Fullness level: 1 2 3 4 5
....

LUNCH
Time .... am/pm ....   Hunger level: 1 2 3 4 5
Hunger cue: ....
What do I want? ....
What and where did I eat? ....
....
....
How do I feel? ....   Fullness level: 1 2 3 4 5
....

SNACK
Time .... am/pm ....   Hunger level: 1 2 3 4 5
Hunger cue: ....
What do I want? ....
What and where did I eat? ....
....
....
How do I feel? ....   Fullness level: 1 2 3 4 5
....

FRUITS AND VEGGIES:

DINNER

Time .... am/pm .... Hunger level: **1 2 3 4 5**

Hunger cue: ....

What do I want? ....

What and where did I eat? ....

....

....

How do I feel? .... Fullness level: **1 2 3 4 5**

....

SNACK

Time .... am/pm .... Hunger level: **1 2 3 4 5**

Hunger cue: ....

What do I want? ....

What and where did I eat? ....

....

....

How do I feel? .... Fullness level: **1 2 3 4 5**

....

EXERCISE

Time .... am/pm

How did I feel before? ....

....

Activity performed: ....

....

....

How do I feel after? ....

....

WATER: 🥤 🥤 🥤 🥤 🥤 🥤 🥤 🥤

UNCOVER THE MEANING OF YOUR CRAVINGS

Honor your body by listening to your cravings and supplying your body with the nutrients you may be in search of. Sometimes your body craves specific foods as a result of lacking certain minerals, vitamins, and other nutrients. To combat these cravings you can try to supply your body with healthy sources of the missing (or low-level) nutrients. On the opposite page are some common cravings, the nutrients associated with them that you may actually be craving, and healthy alternative sources. However, this does not mean cravings are *always* based on a nutrient deficiency. In many cases you may want to eat a cupcake because you want a sweet, not because you are lacking phosphorous. But it's helpful to take note of these cravings to see if you can notice any patterns and address any nutrient deficiencies that you may have.

ACTIVITY OF THE DAY

Monitor you cravings for the day and try to decipher if you are craving for nutritional reasons or not. Record your findings below.

....

....

....

....

....

Are you craving?	You may be lacking ...	Try eating this!
Alcohol	Protein	Meat, poultry, nuts, seafood
	Avenin	Granola, oatmeal
	Calcium	Broccoli, kale, cheese, legumes
Bread/Carbs	Nitrogen	Fish, meat, nuts, beans
Chocolate	Magnesium	Spinach, nuts, seeds, legumes, fruit
Coffee/Tea	Phosphorous	Chicken, beef, poultry, eggs, dairy, nuts, legumes
	Sulfur	Egg yolks, red peppers, onion
	Iron	Meat, seaweed, spinach
Oily Snacks	Calcium	Broccoli, milk, mustard and turnip greens
Salty Foods	Sodium chloride	Sea salt, raw goat milk, nuts
Soda/Carbonated Drinks	Calcium	Broccoli, milk, legumes, cheese, dark leafy greens
Sugar/Sweets	Chromium	Grapes, cheese, broccoli
	Carbon	Fresh fruits
	Phosphorus	Chicken, beef, poultry, eggs, nuts, dairy
	Sulfur	Cranberries, cabbage, kale

When you truly understand that your food choices are powerful and life-affirming, you can exercise control and restraint without deprivation.

MARLETE ADELMANN

DATE:	M	T	W	Th	F	S	Su

BREAKFAST

Time _____ am/pm   Hunger level: 1 2 3 4 5

Hunger cue: _____

What do I want? _____

What and where did I eat? _____

_____

How do I feel? _____   Fullness level: 1 2 3 4 5

_____

LUNCH

Time _____ am/pm   Hunger level: 1 2 3 4 5

Hunger cue: _____

What do I want? _____

What and where did I eat? _____

_____

How do I feel? _____   Fullness level: 1 2 3 4 5

_____

SNACK

Time _____ am/pm   Hunger level: 1 2 3 4 5

Hunger cue: _____

What do I want? _____

What and where did I eat? _____

_____

How do I feel? _____   Fullness level: 1 2 3 4 5

_____

FRUITS AND VEGGIES:

DINNER

Time _____ am/pm   Hunger level: 1 2 3 4 5

Hunger cue:

What do I want?

What and where did I eat?

How do I feel? _____   Fullness level: 1 2 3 4 5

SNACK

Time _____ am/pm   Hunger level: 1 2 3 4 5

Hunger cue:

What do I want?

What and where did I eat?

How do I feel? _____   Fullness level: 1 2 3 4 5

EXERCISE

Time _____ am/pm

How did I feel before?

Activity performed:

How do I feel after?

WATER: 🥛 🥛 🥛 🥛 🥛 🥛 🥛 🥛

EXERCISE INTUITIVELY

Exercise is a gift for the body, not a punishment. Rest when it is required, but identify the difference between needing a rest vs. feeling lethargic, in which case getting out for a walk or a swim could be just the thing you need to feel invigorated! Exercise releases endorphins into your body, which produce positive feelings. Try to find exercises that you enjoy doing, such as yoga, rowing, or even online classes. As with food, it is the exercise choices you make consistently that create well being.

Incorporate exercise into your daily life, in simple ways such as:
• Playing with your pet
• Taking the stairs
• Parking further away
• Walking on your lunch break
• Calf raises while waiting in line or brushing your teeth
• Gentle stretching in your bed before or after sleep

FIND YOUR INTUITIVE EXERCISE STYLE QUIZ
The purpose of this quiz is to give you insight into what type of exercise you enjoy and even thrive from. As with your eating journey you may notice that your intuitive exercise style changes. Feel free to come back to this quiz at any time to reassess where you're at.

1. What type of activity appeals to you the most?
a. Bike riding
b. Lifting weights
c. Boot camp

2. At work you tend to…
a. Work from home and have a flexible schedule.
b. Start and end at the same time each day.
c. Enjoy talking to colleagues rather than doing paperwork.

3. On a Friday night you will most likely be found...

a. On a road trip.

b. Doing what you typically do each weekend.

c. Going out with your closest friends.

4. Your ideal day looks like...

a. Doing whatever you please in the moment.

b. Waking up. Reading the newspaper. Going for a jog with the dog. Going out for lunch. Doing some shopping. Relaxing in the bath with a book.

c. Going out with friends and family for activities and delicious meals.

5. Your favorite meal is...

a. You can't pick a favorite. You like to try new things as often as you can!

b. Steak and potatoes.

c. Spent around the dinner table with your family.

IF YOU GOT:

Mostly A's...You're likely a free spirit. You like to change things up and try new things. Honoring your body to you means that you constantly change your activities. Here is a list of activities to inspire you: mountain biking, rock climbing, hiking, yoga, participating in a mud run, or parkour.

Mostly B's...You're likely a gym junkie. You feel your best when you are following a regimented routine. If you are not already, you may benefit from joining a local gym and setting your alarm to attend daily.

Mostly C's...You're likely a social butterfly. You thrive in group activities and feel your best when you are connecting with others while exercising. Try meeting your best friend for walks, join group fitness classes, attend a yoga class, or join a cycling club.

ACTIVITY OF THE DAY

Exercise intuitively. If you hate running, do not go for a run. Instead, try something that excites you. After completing the quiz above look at your results for some inspiration to get your body moving today!

BREAKFAST

Time _____ am/pm   Hunger level: **1** 2 3 4 5

Hunger cue: _____

What do I want? _____

What and where did I eat? _____

_____

How do I feel? _____ Fullness level: **1** 2 3 4 5

_____

LUNCH

Time _____ am/pm   Hunger level: **1** 2 3 4 5

Hunger cue: _____

What do I want? _____

What and where did I eat? _____

_____

How do I feel? _____ Fullness level: **1** 2 3 4 5

_____

SNACK

Time _____ am/pm   Hunger level: **1** 2 3 4 5

Hunger cue: _____

What do I want? _____

What and where did I eat? _____

_____

How do I feel? _____ Fullness level: **1** 2 3 4 5

_____

FRUITS AND VEGGIES:

DINNER

Time .... am/pm .... Hunger level: **1 2 3 4 5**

Hunger cue: ....

What do I want? ....

What and where did I eat? ....

....

....

How do I feel? .... Fullness level: **1 2 3 4 5**

....

SNACK

Time .... am/pm .... Hunger level: **1 2 3 4 5**

Hunger cue: ....

What do I want? ....

What and where did I eat? ....

....

....

How do I feel? .... Fullness level: **1 2 3 4 5**

....

EXERCISE

Time .... am/pm ....

How did I feel before? ....

....

Activity performed: ....

....

....

How do I feel after? ....

....

WATER: 🥤 🥤 🥤 🥤 🥤 🥤 🥤 🥤

STOP USING FOOD AS YOUR THERAPIST

*Being extremely honest with oneself
is a good exercise.*

SIGMUND FREUD

People tend to use food, or lack thereof, as an escape route from feelings, to-do lists, or problems. In essence, food can become their chosen "therapy." Rather than dealing with whatever emotions they may be feeling, they distract themselves from those feelings with food *(see Emotion-Driven Eating on page 24)*. Unfortunately, food does not fix problems or feelings—it only serves as a distraction.

When you are faced with the temptation to eat in order to combat whatever emotions you may be feeling at a specific time, it's helpful to utilize short-term coping mechanisms such as calling an old friend, intuitively exercising, or trying one of the mindful activities you came up with on Day 5 *(see page 20)*. But it's also important to think long-term. Each emotion we have has its own trigger, and each has its own solution. The key is getting in touch with your emotions. It's not an easy task and won't happen overnight, but begin to think about ways in which you can become more in touch with your feelings. This may include going to a therapist, or finding ways to express yourself creatively—everyone will have a different path. The further you explore this path, the closer you will come to having the ability to confront your emotions head-on, rather than repressing them with food. When you uncover your emotions you can start to create a more loving environment for your body by creating healthy boundaries with yourself and others. Remember that your boundaries will constantly change as your feelings do, which is why mindfulness is such an important tool to honor your body—no one knows your feelings better than you!

ACTIVITY OF THE DAY

With your increasing insight and mindfulness, you can identify your feelings of loneliness or stress and practice sitting with your emotions. With this difficult but rewarding technique you will learn to tell yourself it is okay to feel your emotions—you do not have to change them. This helps you to develop an understanding of your emotions and an unconditional love for yourself. Although it may be uncomfortable at first, sitting with your emotions becomes easier with practice.

"Feel Your Feelings" Technique

First, find a quiet, comfortable spot without any distractions. Use a pillow or padded cushion if you're sitting on the floor. You may also sit in a chair. Close your eyes and take a few deep breaths. Be aware of any emotions you may be feeling. Whatever they are, tell yourself that it is okay to feel them. You have the right to feel whatever you are feeling—without any judgment or guilt. As you become aware of an emotion, recognize and identify it. Acknowledge your feeling and know that you have the power to choose to stay in this emotion or choose to intentionally release this emotion. Whichever you choose, continue to sit and feel how you feel—connecting to the body and breath for a few more minutes.

DATE: M   T   W   Th   F   S   Su

BREAKFAST

Time _____ am/pm _____   Hunger level: **1** 2 3 4 5

Hunger cue: _____

What do I want? _____

What and where did I eat? _____

_____

_____

How do I feel? _____   Fullness level: **1** 2 3 4 5

LUNCH

Time _____ am/pm _____   Hunger level: **1** 2 3 4 5

Hunger cue: _____

What do I want? _____

What and where did I eat? _____

_____

_____

How do I feel? _____   Fullness level: **1** 2 3 4 5

SNACK

Time _____ am/pm _____   Hunger level: **1** 2 3 4 5

Hunger cue: _____

What do I want? _____

What and where did I eat? _____

_____

_____

How do I feel? _____   Fullness level: **1** 2 3 4 5

FRUITS AND VEGGIES:

DINNER

Time .... am/pm .... Hunger level: **1 2 3 4 5**

Hunger cue: ....

What do I want? ....

What and where did I eat? ....

....

....

How do I feel? .... Fullness level: **1 2 3 4 5**

....

SNACK

Time .... am/pm .... Hunger level: **1 2 3 4 5**

Hunger cue: ....

What do I want? ....

What and where did I eat? ....

....

....

How do I feel? .... Fullness level: **1 2 3 4 5**

....

EXERCISE

Time .... am/pm ....

How did I feel before? ....

....

Activity performed: ....

....

....

How do I feel after? ....

....

WATER: 🥤 🥤 🥤 🥤 🥤 🥤 🥤 🥤

INTUITIVE EATER VS. DIET MENTALITY

Consider the chart below. Do any of these questions and descriptions sound familiar? Which statements do you find yourself identifying with?

INTUITIVE EATER	DIET MENTALITY
Am I hungry?	Do I deserve to eat this? Am I allowed to eat again?
Will it be satisfying?	Is there something with fewer calories?
Does it taste good?	How much can I eat? Is it healthy?
Eating is a pleasurable experience.	Eating must be monitored or I will gain weight. Eating is a scheduled routine.
I can celebrate my birthday and eat my cake too.	I cannot celebrate because I cannot eat cake. I am afraid to go to parties because there are too many tempting foods.
I focus on how I feel during excercise. I exercise to feel good.	Exercise is a chore. I exercise to lose weight.
Weight is a number.	My self-worth is based upon my weight.
I listen to my body.	I listen to what the media tells me to eat. I eat based on what time I am supposed to eat.
I trust my body.	I cannot keep unhealthy food in the house because I will eat everything. I need to count calories or I will be overweight.

If you find yourself identifying with the INTUITIVE EATER...

Congratulations! You are almost done with this journal, though the journey has just begun. You have learned the basic principles of intuitive eating and can carry them with you throughout your life wherever you go.

If you find yourself identifying with the DIET MENTALITY...

Congratulations! You have taken the first step to transforming your eating patterns. Now that you have identified your mind-set, you can choose to shift your mentality to listen to your body. Trust me, I know it can take some time to shift your mind-set if you have been living this way for some time—try to have patience with yourself. I recommend continuing to keep track of your intuitive eating journey, this time remembering your "why" for starting this journey and staying committed to shifting your perception toward food.

Everybody has mental chatter—what matters most is becoming aware of what that chatter is saying. When you harness your awareness and notice the story you tell yourself, often you will uncover whether you are living intuitively or stuck living "in lack" with a diet mentality. Remember that what you align yourself with is what you will attract more of in your life.

Live life as if everything is
rigged in your favor.
RUMI

ACTIVITY OF THE DAY

Make a Vision Board for a Mindful Life

Materials Needed:

- Bulletin board
- Paper
- Affirmations, quotes
- Inspiring items that can fit on your board
- Tape, push pins
- Markers
- Photographs, magazine cutouts

A vision board displays your dreams, goals, and optimal life. Focusing on pictures, quotes, and other items you place on your vision board creates a powerful intention to live the life of your dreams.

Choose photographs, images, and quotes that inspire you to think and feel positive. Arrange them on your bulletin board.

Each morning and night spend some time looking at your board and visualizing your mindful life. As time goes by, you will begin to notice your aspirations manifesting. Once your dreams are manifesting you can update your vision board as your life evolves.

- Look at your vision board often.

- Read your affirmations and quotes aloud, with intention.

- Visualize yourself living mindfully.

- Think about what you are grateful for in your life already and write it down on the next page.

What I am grateful for:

DATE: M T W Th F S Su

BREAKFAST

Time .... am/pm .... Hunger level: 1 2 3 4 5

Hunger cue: ....

What do I want? ....

What and where did I eat? ....

....

....

How do I feel? .... Fullness level: 1 2 3 4 5

....

LUNCH

Time .... am/pm .... Hunger level: 1 2 3 4 5

Hunger cue: ....

What do I want? ....

What and where did I eat? ....

....

....

How do I feel? .... Fullness level: 1 2 3 4 5

....

SNACK

Time .... am/pm .... Hunger level: 1 2 3 4 5

Hunger cue: ....

What do I want? ....

What and where did I eat? ....

....

....

How do I feel? .... Fullness level: 1 2 3 4 5

....

FRUITS AND VEGGIES:

DINNER

Time .... am/pm   Hunger level: **1 2 3 4 5**

Hunger cue: ....

What do I want? ....

What and where did I eat? ....

....

....

How do I feel? ....   Fullness level: **1 2 3 4 5**

....

SNACK

Time .... am/pm   Hunger level: **1 2 3 4 5**

Hunger cue: ....

What do I want? ....

What and where did I eat? ....

....

....

How do I feel? ....   Fullness level: **1 2 3 4 5**

....

EXERCISE

Time .... am/pm

How did I feel before? ....

....

Activity performed: ....

....

....

How do I feel after? ....

....

WATER: ⬤ ⬤ ⬤ ⬤ ⬤ ⬤ ⬤ ⬤

EMBRACING YOUR INTUITION

In•tu•i•tion
[in-too-ish-uhn]

"A natural ability or power that makes it possible to know something without any proof or evidence."

Living an intuitive life allows you to nourish your body, mind, and soul. Just like intuitive eating, intuitive living is a practice of doing what feels natural for you. Intuitive living can be hard in our society, but every moment you have a chance to honor your intuition and follow your joy. Give yourself unconditional permission to honor your feelings, sleep cycle, and eating habits.

Congratulations on finishing the *21-Day Workbook & Journal for Intuitive Eating*! You've persevered through the daily activities, cultivated acceptance for where you are in this moment, and may have gone through many ups and downs through the journey to develop an understanding of your body. Take what you've learned in this workbook and continue to explore, learn, and listen to your intuition daily to live a life filled with joy! Take a moment to feel some gratitude toward yourself for picking up this book and continually choosing to honor and nourish yourself every single day. This is a milestone in your life. You are now living free from food compulsions so make sure to treat yourself to some loving self-care today. Revisit this workbook as often as you need to remind yourself how far you've come.

I'd love to hear your story and how this journal has changed your life! Connect with me through:

Instagram: gillianelizab3th
Email: gillianelizabethwc@gmail.com
Facebook: www.facebook.com/gillianelizab3th

ACTIVITY OF THE DAY

Meditation has been mentioned a few times within this program as a way to become more in tune with yourself and also to increase your mindfulness. Today's challenge is to practice meditation for at least 10 minutes. You can individualize the experience by choosing to practice in a way that suits you; you may sit or lie down, you may listen to a guided meditation or enjoy the silence. Attempt to integrate this into your life and carry this practice forward.

You may be in the same boat as many others and think that there is a particular way to meditate and worry that you're not doing it correctly. Let's get one thing straight—there's no right or wrong way to meditate! Phew! Now that we've established that, use the **Meditation 101 Guidelines** *(see page 94)* for some tips.

DATE:	M T W Th F S Su

BREAKFAST

Time .... am/pm .... Hunger level: 1 2 3 4 5

Hunger cue: ....

What do I want? ....

What and where did I eat? ....

....

....

How do I feel? .... Fullness level: 1 2 3 4 5

....

LUNCH

Time .... am/pm .... Hunger level: 1 2 3 4 5

Hunger cue: ....

What do I want? ....

What and where did I eat? ....

....

....

How do I feel? .... Fullness level: 1 2 3 4 5

....

SNACK

Time .... am/pm .... Hunger level: 1 2 3 4 5

Hunger cue: ....

What do I want? ....

What and where did I eat? ....

....

....

How do I feel? .... Fullness level: 1 2 3 4 5

....

FRUITS AND VEGGIES:

DINNER

Time .... am/pm   Hunger level: **1 2 3 4 5**

Hunger cue: ....

What do I want? ....

What and where did I eat? ....

....

....

How do I feel? ....   Fullness level: **1 2 3 4 5**

....

SNACK

Time .... am/pm   Hunger level: **1 2 3 4 5**

Hunger cue: ....

What do I want? ....

What and where did I eat? ....

....

....

How do I feel? ....   Fullness level: **1 2 3 4 5**

....

EXERCISE

Time .... am/pm

How did I feel before? ....

....

Activity performed: ....

....

....

How do I feel after? ....

WATER: 🥛 🥛 🥛 🥛 🥛 🥛 🥛 🥛

MEDITATION 101 GUIDELINES

1. **How to position my body?** Always get into a comfortable position, whether lying down or sitting with a straight spine. Maybe cover yourself with a blanket if you get cold easily. I like to lay in bed on my back as if in savasana pose with the blanket over me, though you have to find what works for you. (Some people find this position too difficult to lay in without falling asleep!)

2. **Where should I meditate?** You can meditate anywhere you feel comfortable—inside or outside. Never meditate while driving. (You should be closing your eyes while you meditate and focus solely on going inward.) A lot of people have the misconception that you need quiet around you to meditate. Yes, this certainly encourages a more focused practice, but if you hear construction outside or your phone is going off, see it as an opportunity to challenge yourself and cultivate your attention even more.

3. **How long do I meditate?** Typically, I recommend meditating for half an hour in the morning and half an hour in the evening. If sitting for half an hour seems like a daunting task, start with 5 minutes and work your way up in increments as you feel ready. Some days it can take the entire 30 minutes to quiet the mind, which is why it's important to give yourself the time to sit for as long as needed. I've even recommended taking "one-minute miracles" to some of my clients who feel overwhelmed by the thought of sitting for so long. Try to take one minute when you wake up and before you go to bed to check in with yourself.

4. **Am I supposed to have no thoughts?** If you're having a lot of racing thoughts you can try to limit the variety by envisioning the word "In" when you inhale and "Out" when you exhale. It's important to remember that the goal isn't to have no thoughts but rather to become aware when you're having a thought and then to bring your attention back to the breath, staying present with yourself. Namaste.

There is something in every one of you that
waits and listens for the sound of the genuine in
yourself. It is the only true guide you will ever have.
And if you cannot hear it, you will all of
your life spend your days on the ends of
strings that somebody else pulls.

HOWARD THURMAN

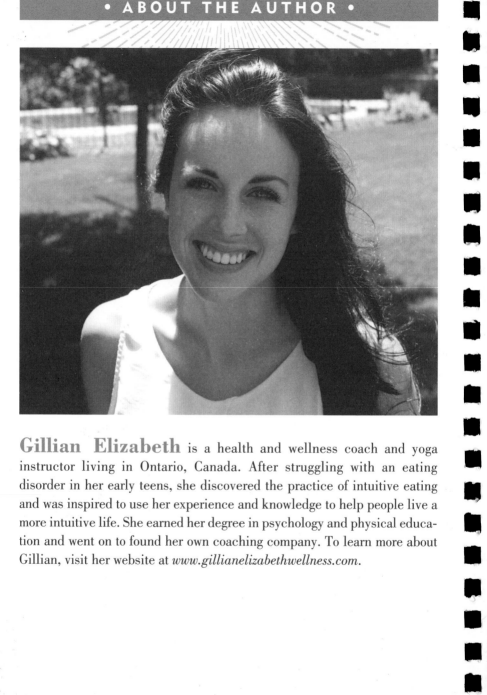

Gillian Elizabeth is a health and wellness coach and yoga instructor living in Ontario, Canada. After struggling with an eating disorder in her early teens, she discovered the practice of intuitive eating and was inspired to use her experience and knowledge to help people live a more intuitive life. She earned her degree in psychology and physical education and went on to found her own coaching company. To learn more about Gillian, visit her website at *www.gillianelizabethwellness.com*.